The Prostate Cancer Kitchen:

Nourishing Recipes for Women Supporting Loved Ones Through Treatment

By

Elizabeth J. Gallagher

Table of contents

Introduction

Welcome to "The Prostate Cancer Kitchen: Nourishing Recipes for Women Supporting Loved Ones Through Treatment." This cookbook is designed for the women who are supporting their partners, family members, or friends through prostate cancer treatment. Prostate cancer can be a challenging and overwhelming experience, not only for the individual undergoing treatment but also for the caregiver. One important aspect of managing prostate cancer is a healthy diet. A balanced and nutrient-rich diet can help support the body during treatment and recovery.

This cookbook offers a variety of delicious and healthy recipes that incorporate prostate cancer-fighting foods such as fruits, vegetables, whole grains, lean proteins, and healthy fats. The recipes are easy to follow and are designed to help you make healthier choices while still enjoying tasty and satisfying meals. Whether you're looking for breakfast, lunch, dinner, or snack ideas, this cookbook has something for everyone.

In addition to recipes, this cookbook also offers tips for meal planning, grocery shopping, and cooking techniques. You'll find information on ingredient substitutions, eating out, and how to incorporate prostate cancer-fighting foods into your diet in a variety of ways. The goal of this cookbook is to empower women supporting loved ones through prostate cancer treatment to make healthy and delicious meals that support their health and wellbeing.

Remember, a healthy diet is just one part of managing prostate cancer. Always consult with a healthcare professional to ensure that you're following an appropriate diet for your individual needs and circumstances. We hope that this cookbook can provide you with inspiration and support as you navigate the challenges of prostate cancer treatment.

Chapter 1: Understanding Prostate Cancer

Prostate cancer is the most common cancer among men worldwide. While it is a serious disease, there are ways to manage it effectively, including through changes in diet and lifestyle. This book is a comprehensive guide to eating well during and after prostate cancer treatment. By providing practical advice and delicious recipes, we hope to support those with prostate cancer in making informed choices about their diet and nutrition.

Prostate Cancer: An Overview

The prostate is a gland in the male reproductive system that produces fluid to nourish and transport sperm. Prostate cancer occurs when abnormal cells in the prostate gland begin to grow uncontrollably. While some cases of prostate cancer may not cause symptoms, others may cause urinary problems, pain, or other symptoms.

Risk Factors for Prostate Cancer

While the exact cause of prostate cancer is not known, there are several risk factors that may increase a man's likelihood of developing the disease. These include:

1. Age: Prostate cancer is more common in older men, with the majority of cases occurring in men over the age of 65.
2. Family history: Men with a family history of prostate cancer may be at increased risk of developing the disease.
3. Race: African American men are more likely to develop prostate cancer than men of other races.
4. Diet and lifestyle: A diet high in red meat and processed foods, as well as a sedentary lifestyle, may increase the risk of developing prostate cancer.

In this book, you'll find evidence-based information about the role of diet in prostate cancer treatment, as well as tips for creating balanced meals that can help you maintain your strength and support your immune system. We've also included recipes that are easy to prepare and delicious to eat, so you can enjoy your meals while feeling good about what you're putting into your body.

Whether you're newly diagnosed with prostate cancer or a long-time survivor, this book can help you make choices that support your health and wellbeing. By following the advice and recipes within these pages, you can feel confident that you're doing everything you can to support your body during this challenging time. So let's get started!

Chapter 2: Why Diet Matters in Prostate Cancer Treatment

Prostate cancer is a complex disease, and there is no one-size-fits-all approach to treatment. However, research has shown that diet can play an important role in supporting prostate cancer treatment and recovery. In this chapter, we'll explore some of the reasons why diet matters in prostate cancer treatment.

First and foremost, a healthy diet can help you maintain your strength and energy levels, which is important during and after prostate cancer treatment. Cancer and cancer treatment can take a toll on your body, and eating well can help you stay as strong and healthy as possible.

In addition, some foods have been shown to have specific benefits for prostate cancer patients. For example, foods that are high in antioxidants, such as fruits and vegetables, can help protect your cells from damage and support your immune system. Similarly, foods that are high in fiber, such as whole grains and legumes, can help regulate your digestive system and reduce inflammation in the body.

On the other hand, some foods and nutrients may have negative effects on prostate cancer treatment. For example, a diet high in saturated fat may increase inflammation in the body, which can make cancer treatment less effective. Similarly, excess alcohol consumption can increase your risk of developing certain types of cancer, including prostate cancer.

Overall, diet is an important part of prostate cancer treatment and recovery. By making informed choices about what you eat, you can support your body's natural healing processes and improve your overall quality of life. In the next chapter, we'll explore some of the specific foods that can help support prostate cancer treatment.

Chapter 3: The Importance of a Balanced Diet

Eating a balanced diet is important for everyone, but it is especially important for prostate cancer patients. A balanced diet can help you maintain your strength and energy levels, support your immune system, and reduce your risk of developing other health problems.

So, what is a balanced diet? Simply put, a balanced diet is one that includes a variety of different foods from all the major food groups. These include:

1. Fruits and vegetables: Aim to eat at least five servings of fruits and vegetables every day. These foods are high in antioxidants, which can help protect your cells from damage.

2. Whole grains: Whole grains are an important source of fiber, which can help regulate your digestive system and reduce inflammation in the body. Examples of whole grains include whole wheat, brown rice, quinoa, and oatmeal.

3. Lean protein: Choose lean sources of protein, such as chicken, fish, beans, and tofu. These foods are

important for maintaining muscle mass and repairing tissues.

3. Low-fat dairy: Dairy products are an important source of calcium, which is essential for maintaining strong bones. Choose low-fat options, such as skim milk, low-fat cheese, and yogurt.

4. Healthy fats: Include healthy fats in your diet, such as olive oil, nuts, and seeds. These foods can help reduce inflammation in the body and support your heart health.

In addition to including these foods in your diet, it's also important to limit your intake of processed foods, sugary drinks, and foods that are high in saturated and trans fats. These foods can increase inflammation in the body and make cancer treatment less effective.

By eating a balanced diet that includes a variety of different foods, you can support your body's natural healing processes and improve your overall quality of life. In the next chapter, we'll explore some of the specific foods that can be especially beneficial for prostate cancer patients.

Chapter 4: Foods to Include in Your Diet

When it comes to eating well during and after prostate cancer treatment, there are a number of foods that can be especially beneficial. In this chapter, we'll explore some of the foods that you should consider including in your diet.

1. Cruciferous vegetables: Vegetables such as broccoli, cauliflower, kale, and Brussels sprouts are high in compounds called glucosinolates, which have been shown to have anti-cancer properties.

2. Tomatoes: Tomatoes are high in lycopene, a powerful antioxidant that may help protect against prostate cancer.

3. Berries: Berries are high in antioxidants, which can help protect your cells from damage. They are also a good source of fiber.

4. Green tea: Green tea is high in antioxidants called catechins, which may help protect against cancer.

5. Fish: Fatty fish, such as salmon and tuna, are high in omega-3 fatty acids, which have anti-inflammatory properties and may help reduce your risk of developing prostate cancer.

6. Legumes: Legumes, such as beans, lentils, and chickpeas, are a good source of protein and fiber. They also contain compounds called phytoestrogens, which have been shown to have anti-cancer properties.

7. Whole grains: Whole grains, such as brown rice and quinoa, are a good source of fiber and may help reduce inflammation in the body.

8. Nuts and seeds: Nuts and seeds, such as almonds, walnuts, and flaxseed, are a good source of healthy fats and may help reduce inflammation in the body.

By including these foods in your diet, you can support your body's natural healing processes and reduce your risk of developing other health problems. In the next chapter, we'll explore some of the foods that you should limit or avoid during prostate cancer treatment.

Chapter 5: Foods to Limit or Avoid During Prostate Cancer Treatment

While there are many foods that can be beneficial during prostate cancer treatment, there are also some foods that you should limit or avoid. In this chapter, we'll explore some of the foods that you should be cautious about consuming.

1. Red and processed meats: Red and processed meats, such as beef, pork, hot dogs, and bacon, are high in saturated fats and may increase inflammation in the body. Research

has also linked high consumption of red and processed meats to an increased risk of developing prostate cancer.

2. Dairy products: While dairy products are an important source of calcium, some research has suggested that high consumption of dairy products may increase your risk of developing prostate cancer.

3. Sugar and sugary drinks: Foods that are high in sugar, such as candy, soda, and baked goods, may increase inflammation in the body and contribute to weight gain.

4.   Alcohol: Excessive alcohol consumption may increase your risk of developing prostate cancer and may also interfere with cancer treatment.

5. Processed foods: Processed foods, such as fast food and pre-packaged meals, are often high in sodium and unhealthy fats. These foods may increase inflammation in the body and contribute to weight gain.

6. Fried foods: Fried foods, such as French fries and fried chicken, are often high in unhealthy fats and may increase inflammation in the body.

While it's important to limit your consumption of these foods, it's also important to maintain a balanced diet that includes a variety of different foods. Talk to your doctor or a registered dietitian to develop a personalized nutrition plan that meets your individual needs.

Chapter 6: Healthy and Delicious Recipes

In this chapter, we'll provide you with some healthy and delicious recipes that you can incorporate into your diet during and after prostate cancer treatment.

1. Broccoli and Tomato Quiche: This recipe is packed with prostate-protective vegetables and makes for a nutritious and filling breakfast or brunch dish.

2. Grilled Salmon with Lemon and Dill: This simple and flavorful dish is packed with omega-3 fatty acids, which have been shown to have

anti-inflammatory properties and may help reduce your risk of developing prostate cancer.

3. Lentil and Vegetable Soup: This hearty and comforting soup is high in fiber, protein, and phytochemicals, which have been shown to have anti-cancer properties.

4. Roasted Brussels Sprouts and Sweet Potatoes: This flavorful and colorful side dish is high in fiber, vitamins, and antioxidants, making it a great addition to any meal.

5. Mixed Berry Smoothie: This refreshing smoothie is packed with antioxidants, fiber, and protein,

making it a nutritious and delicious breakfast or snack option.

6. Black Bean and Vegetable Stir-Fry: This quick and easy stir-fry is packed with protein, fiber, and phytochemicals, making it a nutritious and satisfying meal.

By incorporating these recipes into your diet, you can ensure that you're getting the nutrients your body needs to support your natural healing processes and reduce your risk of developing other health problems. Remember to talk to your doctor or a registered dietitian before making any significant changes to your diet.

Chapter 7: Tips for Meal Planning and Preparation

In this chapter, we'll provide you with some tips for meal planning and preparation to help make healthy eating during prostate cancer treatment easier and more enjoyable.

1. Plan ahead: Take some time each week to plan out your meals and snacks. This will help you ensure that you're getting a variety of different foods and nutrients, and will make it easier to stick to your dietary goals.

2. Shop smart: When you're grocery shopping, stick to the perimeter of the store, where the fresh fruits, vegetables, and lean proteins are located. Avoid the processed and packaged foods in the center aisles as much as possible.

3. Cook in batches: Cook large batches of healthy meals and freeze them in individual portions. This will make it easy to have a healthy meal on hand when you're short on time or not feeling up to cooking.

4. Make use of leftovers: Don't let leftovers go to waste! Use them to create new meals, such as turning leftover grilled chicken into a chicken

salad or adding leftover vegetables to a soup or stir-fry.

5. Use healthy cooking methods: Choose healthy cooking methods, such as grilling, baking, or steaming, instead of frying or sautéing in unhealthy fats.

6. Make healthy swaps: Look for ways to make healthier swaps in your favorite recipes, such as using whole wheat pasta instead of regular pasta or using Greek yogurt instead of sour cream.

7. Stay hydrated: Drink plenty of water throughout the day to stay

hydrated and help flush toxins out of your body.

By following these tips for meal planning and preparation, you can make healthy eating during prostate cancer treatment easier and more enjoyable. Remember to listen to your body and talk to your doctor or a registered dietitian if you have any questions or concerns about your diet.

Chapter 8: Dining Out and Traveling Tips

In this chapter, we'll provide you with some tips for dining out and traveling while maintaining a healthy diet during prostate cancer treatment.

1. Plan ahead: Before going out to eat or traveling, do some research on healthy dining options in the area. Look for restaurants that offer healthy options, or that are willing to make modifications to their menu to accommodate your dietary needs.

2. Stick to your dietary goals: Don't be afraid to ask your server for modifications to your meal, such as

swapping out unhealthy sides for vegetables or asking for dressing on the side. Stick to your dietary goals as much as possible, even when dining out or traveling.

3. Bring healthy snacks: When traveling, bring along healthy snacks, such as fruit, nuts, or energy bars, to avoid the temptation of unhealthy fast food options.

4. Avoid excessive alcohol consumption: While it's okay to enjoy a drink or two while dining out or on vacation, excessive alcohol consumption can have negative effects on your health and may

increase your risk of developing prostate cancer.

5. Keep portion sizes in check: Many restaurants serve oversized portions, which can lead to overeating and weight gain. Consider splitting an entrée with a friend or asking for a to-go container to take home leftovers.

6. Be mindful of food allergies: If you have any food allergies or intolerances, be sure to communicate this to your server or hotel staff when dining out or traveling.

By following these tips for dining out and traveling while maintaining a healthy diet during prostate cancer treatment, you can stay on track with your dietary goals and enjoy your meals and travels to the fullest. Remember to talk to your doctor or a registered dietitian if you have any questions or concerns about your diet or dietary restrictions.

Chapter 9: Supplement and Vitamin Recommendations

In this chapter, we'll provide you with some recommendations for supplements and vitamins that may be beneficial during prostate cancer treatment.

1. Vitamin D: Vitamin D is important for overall health and may be beneficial for prostate cancer patients. Talk to your doctor or a registered dietitian to determine if a vitamin D supplement is right for you.

2. Omega-3 fatty acids: Omega-3 fatty acids have anti-inflammatory properties and may be beneficial for prostate cancer patients. Consider incorporating sources of omega-3s into your diet, such as fatty fish like salmon, or taking a fish oil supplement.

3. Probiotics: Probiotics are good bacteria that can help improve gut health and boost the immune system. Consider incorporating probiotic-rich foods into your diet, such as yogurt, kefir, or kimchi, or taking a probiotic supplement.

4. Zinc: Zinc is important for overall health and may be beneficial for

prostate cancer patients. Consider incorporating sources of zinc into your diet, such as oysters, beef, or pumpkin seeds, or taking a zinc supplement.

5. Selenium: Selenium is a mineral that may have anti-cancer properties and may be beneficial for prostate cancer patients. Consider incorporating sources of selenium into your diet, such as Brazil nuts, tuna, or chicken, or taking a selenium supplement.

6. Green tea extract: Green tea extract contains antioxidants that may have anti-cancer properties and may be beneficial for prostate cancer patients.

Consider incorporating green tea into your diet or taking a green tea extract supplement.

7. Curcumin: Curcumin is a compound found in turmeric that has anti-inflammatory properties and may have anti-cancer effects. Consider incorporating turmeric into your cooking or taking a curcumin supplement.

8. Vitamin E: Vitamin E is an antioxidant that may have anti-cancer properties and may be beneficial for prostate cancer patients. Consider incorporating sources of vitamin E into your diet, such as almonds,

spinach, or avocados, or taking a vitamin E supplement.

9. Lycopene: Lycopene is a compound found in tomatoes that may have anti-cancer properties and may be beneficial for prostate cancer patients. Consider incorporating tomatoes or tomato products into your diet, such as tomato sauce or canned tomatoes, or taking a lycopene supplement.

10. Melatonin: Melatonin is a hormone that helps regulate sleep and may have anti-cancer properties. Consider taking a melatonin supplement to help improve sleep

quality and potentially benefit your prostate cancer treatment.

Remember that supplements and vitamins should never replace a healthy diet and lifestyle, and should always be taken under the guidance of a healthcare professional. Always talk to your doctor or a registered dietitian before starting any new supplement or vitamin regimen, as some supplements may interact with certain medications or medical conditions. A balanced diet with a variety of nutrient-rich foods is always the best way to support your overall health and wellbeing during prostate cancer treatment.

Chapter 10: Meal Planning and Recipes

In this chapter, we'll provide you with tips for meal planning and some delicious recipes to help you incorporate prostate cancer-fighting foods into your diet.

1. Meal planning tips: When planning your meals, aim to incorporate a variety of nutrient-dense foods such as fruits, vegetables, whole grains, lean proteins, and healthy fats. Consider planning your meals ahead of time to help ensure you have healthy options available throughout the week. You can also try batch cooking or meal prepping to save

time and ensure you have healthy options on hand.

2. Recipe ideas: Here are a few recipe ideas to help you get started:

- Quinoa and vegetable stir-fry: Cook quinoa according to package instructions. In a separate pan, sauté a mix of vegetables such as bell peppers, mushrooms, and onions in olive oil. Mix quinoa and vegetables together and season with herbs and spices.

- Grilled salmon with avocado salsa: Brush salmon filets with olive oil and season with salt and pepper. Grill or bake salmon until cooked through. Top with a fresh salsa made with diced avocado, tomato, red onion, and lime juice.

- Lentil soup: In a large pot, sauté onions, garlic, and carrots in olive oil. Add lentils, vegetable broth, canned tomatoes, and a mix of herbs and spices. Simmer until lentils are cooked through.

- Spinach and goat cheese omelet: Whisk together eggs and a splash of milk. In a pan, sauté spinach in olive oil. Add the egg mixture to the pan and cook until set. Add crumbled goat cheese on top and fold over the omelet.

3. Snack ideas: Snacks can be a great way to incorporate prostate cancer-fighting foods into your diet. Here are a few snack ideas to try:

- Greek yogurt with berries and nuts

- Hummus with carrot sticks or whole-grain crackers

- Apple slices with almond butter

- Trail mix with nuts, seeds, and dried fruit.

4. Tips for eating out: Eating out can be a challenge when trying to follow a healthy diet, but there are ways to make healthier choices. Consider choosing grilled or baked options instead of fried, asking for dressings or sauces on the side, and opting for vegetable sides instead of French fries. You can also research the restaurant menu ahead of time to find healthier options and ask your server for recommendations.

5. Cooking techniques: How you cook your food can impact its nutrient content. Consider grilling, baking, or steaming foods instead of frying, as these cooking methods can help preserve nutrient content.

6. Ingredient substitutions: If you're following a recipe and want to make it healthier, consider swapping out ingredients. For example, you can replace white pasta with whole-grain pasta, use Greek yogurt instead of sour cream, or swap out butter for olive oil.

Remember to focus on a balanced diet with a variety of nutrient-rich foods, and to consult with your doctor or a registered dietitian if you have any specific dietary needs or questions. Incorporating prostate cancer-fighting foods into your meals and snacks can help support your overall health and wellbeing during prostate cancer treatment.

Incorporating a healthy diet is an important part of managing prostate cancer. By including prostate cancer-fighting foods such as fruits, vegetables, whole grains, lean proteins, and healthy fats, you can help support your overall health and wellbeing during treatment. Meal planning and recipe ideas can also help you make healthy choices and incorporate these foods into your diet in a tasty and enjoyable way. Remember to always consult with your doctor or a registered dietitian before making any significant changes to your diet, and to adjust your diet to your individual needs and preferences. With a focus on a balanced and nutrient-rich diet, you can take steps to support your health and wellbeing during prostate cancer treatment.